MW00962111

Blood Pressure Solutions

Your Trustworthy Guide To Lowering
Your Blood Pressure And Living A Happy,
Healthy, And Stress Free Life

Published by Digital Superheroes Publications

No part of this book may be reproduced or transmitted in any form or by any means, electronic or mechanical, including photocopying, recording, or by any information storage and retrieval system, without permission in writing from the publisher.

Book Description

Hypertension, or, as it is more commonly known as, high blood pressure, is an incredibly common disease that affects millions of people worldwide. In the United States alone, over 3 million new cases of hypertension are diagnosed every year.

With this number rising at an alarming rate, you can never be too cautious.

Perhaps you have already been diagnosed with hypertension. Perhaps you have been diagnosed with pre-hypertension and you are now wondering what you can do to stop the disease from progressing further. Perhaps you have gone to the pharmacy with a loved one and discovered they are at risk, or that they in fact do have hypertension themselves.

Regardless of what your reason is, you are now looking for answers. You want to know everything there is to know about high blood pressure, and what you can do to bring your blood pressure level back down to a normal range.

So, what do you do? There are pills you can get on, but those are only so effective against a lifestyle that promotes this disease. So, what lifestyle changes can you make that will lower your blood pressure and give you your healthy life back?

That's where this book comes in. In it, I am going to show you exactly what you need to do to lower your blood pressure, get healthy, and eliminate the risks that are associated with hypertension.

Come on this journey with me, be willing to make the changes you need to make, and enjoy a life that is happy, healthy, and hypertension free, guaranteed.

- **Learn everything you need to know about blood pressure and how to lower yours**

- **Make the changes you need to make to reverse your hypertension**

- **Arm yourself with a healthy lifestyle and live a healthy life**

- **And much, much more!**

Contents

Contents

Introduction

You love your salty foods. Popcorn, potato chips, French fries, salted meats – the list goes on and on. You can't get enough of the breakfast foods and the salty goodness that often accompanies them. It's not that you're overweight, not really, at least.

If you were honest with yourself, you know you could get more exercise than you do right now. But hey, you have a lot of other things going on in your life, and no one wants to spend hours sweating it out at the gym anyway.

You're aware that there have been some heart issues in your family line, but everyone who had those issues was a lot older than you. You still have plenty of time in your life before you have to give thought to such things, right?

Or perhaps none of these things describe you. Perhaps you spend your day at the office, trying to make ends meet. Working with this client, visiting with that one. Doing your best to make every office appointment alone. Delegating never has been your strong suit. After all, if you want something done right, you have to do it yourself, don't you?

Or perhaps you have just found out that you are expecting your first child. Or second, or maybe even your third. Happiness is filling your mind and body almost as fast as pregnancy is taking over, and it isn't long before you start to see the wonderful effects of this condition – on the outside of your body.

It's still a mystery as to what is going on inside.

What do these scenarios and situations have in common? What is the one thing about all these people that ties them all together, regardless of age, gender, what they do for a living, or where they are in life?

Blood pressure.

All these people have blood flowing through their veins, just like everyone else on the planet. The difference? All these people are also at high risk for having high blood pressure.

So, what does that mean? How can it be managed? Is high blood pressure something to worry about, can it be treated?

If you have been diagnosed with high blood pressure, or if you are at risk for developing high blood pressure, you likely have all these questions running through your brain and more.

Being faced with high blood pressure can be a scary thing. When you realize all the adverse side effects that can happen and are faced with the severity of the situation, you can start to feel fearful or even start to panic.

Don't worry. Though high blood pressure is no laughing matter, it is something that can be managed, reversed, and even cured with the right lifestyle. And that is what you are going to discover here.

Come with me on a blood pressure journey, and let me show you everything you need to do to lower your blood pressure and bring it back down into a normal range. It's going to take time and some deliberate effort on your part, but trust me, your health is worth it, your family is worth it, and you are worth it.

I am going to help you get through every step of the way, from helping you understand what hypertension is and what causes it, to how you can effectively, and happily change your life for the better. This doesn't have to be a terrible thing that has happened to you. In fact, it could be the best change you have ever made.

This is your chance to grab life by the horns and take control of your health. Are you ready to make the changes you need to make for a healthier you? Are you ready to prove to your family that you want to be there for them in the long hall? Are you ready to get healthy?

Good.

Let's get started.

Chapter 1 – So You Have High Blood Pressure?

You're driving home from the doctor, thinking about what he just said.

"You have hypertension."

The words sound scary enough as they are, but you wonder, *what does that really mean?*

You've heard of blood pressure. Ever since you were a child you had to endure that band being placed around your arm and pumped full of air at every check up. You watched as the needle danced back and forth, then the doctor suddenly took it off and wrote something down, without you really understanding what was going on.

Perhaps you have heard of high blood pressure in older relatives. Your uncle or your grandfather had it. Perhaps one of them even suffered adverse side effects as a result, but it still didn't hit close to home.

After all, health problems – no matter what they are – happen to other people, not to you.

Yet here you are, diagnosed with high blood pressure, and you aren't sure what that even means.

What is hypertension?

As your blood flows through your arteries, it is exuding a certain amount of pressure. Blood pressure is measured using two different numbers. The systolic number is the number on top, and it represents the pressure that is in your arteries during the time your heart contracts.

The bottom number, known as the diastolic number, is the measurement of the pressure that is placed on your arteries when your heart is relaxed.

Normal blood pressure is a measurement that is lower than 120/80 in a healthy adult. Adults with a measurement of 139/89 are known as having pre-hypertension, which means they are at greater risk for developing hypertension, though they aren't there yet.

Any number that is greater than 140/90 are considered to have hypertension.

Though high blood pressure (hypertension) isn't addressed nearly as often as other common diseases, it is, in fact, incredibly important to get it under control, as hypertension is the gateway to a plethora of other problems.

Many people discover they have hypertension when they visit the doctor, although this doesn't have to be the case. If you know and understand the numbers, you can check your own blood pressure for free at many pharmacies. You can even purchase your own pump to check your pressure levels at home, if you choose.

Hypertension is incredibly common, with 3 million new cases in the United States alone every year. It is a highly treatable condition, both by a medical professional as well as at home. It's not whether you have hypertension that is the bad news, it's what you do with it.

Few people who are diagnosed with hypertension or pre-hypertension take their diagnoses as seriously as they ought to. Though it's not a reason to panic, it is a wake up call to live a healthier life.

In the next chapter, I am going to outline for you the risks and diseases that are associated with hypertension, and show you exactly why it's important to get this issue under control as soon as possible.

Chapter 2 – What's The Big Deal?

Odds are you know several people who have high blood pressure. The odds are even greater that several of these people are in your own family. Often, they are older or overweight adults, although hypertension can strike anyone. With this in mind, it can be easy to overlook the severity of the situation, and not take the proper action to get it under control.

However, hypertension has been linked to a variety of other health issues, some of them serious enough they can potentially be fatal.

Though there are evident symptoms of high blood pressure, many people often assume these symptoms are caused by something else, and don't ever get properly diagnosed.

Other times, high blood pressure produces no symptoms at all, so without regular check ups, this condition has been known as the "silent killer."

With that in mind, it's always important to know what symptoms are, and check to see whether you have them. Of course, you should also be checking your own blood pressure on a normal basis, but in addition, watch out for these:

- Headache – could be a moderate headache or could be a migraine. If you have high blood pressure, this will often not go away, or will quickly come back after taking a pain-relieving medication.

- Dizziness – this can happen when you stand up after sitting or lying down, or it can happen out of the blue. If you are suddenly feeling dizzy and don't know why, make an appointment with your doctor.

- Shortness of breath – the inability to breathe properly is never a good sign, and could indicate that something much worse is going on.

- Blurred vision – you might have a hard time waking up in the morning, but if you find that you can't see properly during the day, or suddenly can't see properly when you could a few minutes before, get in touch with your doctor.

- Feelings of pulsations in either your neck or head (or even both) – high blood pressure is caused by the blood putting a lot of pressure on the arteries as it flows, this can sometimes be felt in the head or neck.

- Nausea – is it high blood pressure or is it the flu? It's always best to get checked out.

None of these symptoms are pleasant to experience, and it's easy for them to be ignored or credited to some other insignificant health issue such as a cold or the flu.

However, if left untreated, hypertension can lead to other, far more serious health risks such as:

- Kidney disease – the kidneys are important for filtering blood, balancing electrolytes, and regulating hormones. When they become diseased or damaged, they won't function properly, leading to other serious health problems.

- Stroke – when not enough blood reaches the brain, a stroke results. A stroke often causes paralysis on one side of the body, slurred speech, and could potentially cause death. Those who survive having a stroke are often left to live life with severe disabilities.

- Heart attack – a heart attack results when a blood clot blocks the coronary artery, preventing more blood from reaching the heart, and resulting in the heart muscle dying. Depending on the severity of the attack, and without immediate, expert assistance, heart attacks are almost always fatal.

The first list of symptoms did appear to be uncomfortable, but when you look at the gravity of what hypertension can lead to, you are left with a far more accurate assessment of how serious this condition truly is.

Keep in mind that this isn't an exhaustive list, and there are still other things that can potentially happen from untreated high blood pressure as well. Though the diagnoses in and of itself is nothing to panic about, leaving it untreated is a serious matter.

Let's continue on our journey of understanding what hypertension is, and how you can bring your blood pressure level back down to a normal range, and avoid any and all of these adverse side effects.

Chapter 3 – Is High Blood Pressure a Disease?

Any diagnosis is scary, especially when you don't have the answers. When you hear that you have something that has to be "managed", it's easy to think that you have a disease, and can no longer live a normal life.

When it comes to hypertension, this isn't true. Of course, you do need to make some drastic lifestyle changes that will lower your blood pressure, but you aren't going to have to think about your blood pressure at every moment of every day, or have to give up on doing things because of the fact you have it.

In fact, with high blood pressure, you will be motived to do more things to bring it back down to a manageable level. One of the biggest things you can do for your health at this point is to become more active – meaning finding things you like to do and getting out and doing them.

Now, let's get a greater understanding of blood pressure, and what causes it to become too high.

How is blood pressure measured?

We already looked at what a normal range for blood pressure is (120/80), but you may still have questions on how the doctor arrives at this measurement. First of all, blood pressure is measured using a tool known as a sphygmomanometer – which is that little pump he places around your arm in the examination room.

The pressure is measured in millimeters of mercury, which is why you always see the abbreviation *mm Hg*.

As the doctor pumps the air into the sphygmomanometer, the pressure on your arm also puts pressure on your arteries, and by putting a stethoscope on your arm, the doctor can listen to the sound of the blood being pushed through.

The doctor then calculates the pressure based on what he is hearing, and gives you your results. When you go to the pharmacy, the machine is programmed to measure these pulses through the cuff you put your arm through, giving you an accurate measurement that way as well.

You've already seen the symptoms of high blood pressure, but by now you are no doubt wondering, what causes high blood pressure?

For as common as high blood pressure is in the world today, it is still not entirely certain what causes it exactly. However, there are a number of factors that come into play, and any combination of these factors will greatly increase your risk of developing hypertension in your life.

- Smoking

- Being overweight or obese – it is speculated that the extra weight on a person's body is weighing down on the arteries, causing more pressure to build. Another possible cause is plaque buildup in the walls of the arteries.

- Lack of physical activity – again, without the exertion of physical activity, it is possible that plaque is able to build up within the arteries easier.

- Too much salt in the diet

- Too much alcohol consumption (more than 1 or 2 drinks per day, based on the units of alcohol in the drinks.)

- Stress – stress is a silent killer, and has many adverse side effects on a person's health.

- Older age

- Genetics – though doctors and scientists do not know why, it is evident that high blood pressure, and the problems often associated with high blood pressure, run in families.

- Family history of high blood pressure – again with the genetics.

- Chronic kidney disease – it is unknown in this situation which came first, the disease or the high blood pressure.

- Adrenal or thyroid disorders – again, which came first?

- Sleep apnea

If you take an honest look at this list, odds are you will be able to pick out one or two (or perhaps more) things that you do or have in your life.

Let's face it, we all have stress in our lives, but if you allow stress to build up and never relieve it, you are only setting yourself up for health problems in the future.

Keep in mind – you may have a family history of high blood pressure, and it may be in your genetics, but this is not a reason to give up, nor to think that you are doomed to have it.

Genetics are like the blueprints that help make us who we are. We tend to take on many of the same traits that our parents, and their parents, and their parents had, however, just because there is something in the family line, it does not mean you are going to get it.

Yes, you are predisposed, but doomed? Not at all! Many people give up when they learn that family history is a factor, thinking that they are unable to then break out of the cycle. However, there are so many more things to consider, and so many things you can do to reduce your blood pressure, this doesn't have to be something you are doomed to live with.

With that being said about family history, it's time we take a look at the different risk factor groups that there are.

Perhaps in addition to having a family history you are part of a group which has a higher risk for developing hypertension, or perhaps even without a family history you are part of a group with hypertension. Either way, it is important to understand exactly what your risk factors are, and what you can do to change them.

At the end of the day, some people would consider high blood pressure to be a disease, others would argue that it is merely a condition which needs to be dealt with. The unarguable fact is that if it is left untreated, it most certainly will lead to diseases, and that is what you don't want to happen.

Let's take a look at your particular risk (based on the group you fall in) and how you can adjust what you are doing based on that risk. For some, it is merely a stage of life, for others, they are in need of a lifestyle change.

With no black and white answer to the question, there are certainly some black and white solutions to call on.

Chapter 4 – Find Your Group

High blood pressure, though it is most common seen in people who have the risk factors listed in the last chapter, affects different groups of people differently. As a result, it should be addressed differently, based on the people who are affected. In this chapter, we are going to discuss the different groups of people, and what it means for them to have hypertension.

High blood pressure based on lifestyle choices:

By far the most common group to have high blood pressure are those who have it due to the choices they make in life. As you saw in the last chapter, there are a variety of things you can be doing to contribute to your own high blood pressure, including:

- Bad habits – both smoking and drinking alcohol were on the list. It doesn't matter what you smoke, whether it be cigars, cigarettes, or marijuana medically or recreationally, you are putting yourself at risk for high blood pressure. At the same time, alcohol (regardless of it being beer, wine, or liquor) is also going to put you at risk.

- Diet – a diet that is high in salt is the worst for blood pressure. One of the first things doctors look at after a hypertension diagnosis is what you have been eating.

  It doesn't matter where these salts are coming from – they can be salt you added, highly salted snack foods, processed foods, eating out, salted meats – anything that is adding more salt to your diet is going to raise your blood pressure.

- Stress – as I said, we all have stress in our lives. It's what you do with this stress that matters, and if you have high blood pressure, odds are you aren't dealing with the stress as you ought to be.

  Do things that will relax you. If you have a tough day at the office, go for a run. If you can't seem to get away from the harassing emails, turn off your computer. You are going to deal with stress in your life, but you can't let stress take over your life.

- Inactivity – we all hate those people who love to get up and run, or those people who spend a day at the office, only to head off to the gym for an hour. Yet in all honesty, these people often have normal blood pressure levels.

  Inactivity is a huge factor in causing high blood pressure, as is being overweight (which often stems from diet and inactivity)

So, what can these people do?

The answer is rather obvious. If you are dealing with high blood pressure because of the lifestyle you live, change your lifestyle. Stop adding so much salt to your food, and stop choosing food that is high in salt.

Quit drinking and smoking. You might not be able to imagine a life like that now, but in the long run, it's going to do your health a world of good.

Learn how to reduce stress in a healthy way that leaves you feeling good about yourself. This can be through exercise, meditation, doing something you love, or simply getting away from the pressures of life for a while. Whatever you need to do, do it.

Get active. As you have seen, inactivity is a major player in the world of hypertension, get active and watch not only your blood pressure drop, but the numbers on the scale as well.

High blood pressure in the elderly:

Unfortunately, the older people get, the more likely they are to develop high blood pressure, regardless of the other factors in life. However, as people age, the risk factors for the adverse side effects of high blood pressure also go up.

Though it's relatively normal to hear of an elderly person pass from a heart attack or a stroke, it doesn't have to be this way, and with proper prevention, the elderly can greatly reduce their risk for such things.

Doctors have not spent a lot of time studying why blood pressure is higher in the elderly than it is in younger people, but speculation is that it is because of their arteries becoming worn from age.

However, this doesn't mean that they don't need to take the same precautions as the rest of the world does. And, with these proper precautions, they can greatly reduce their chances of high blood pressure.

When it comes to the elderly, the best thing they can do for their health is through diet and exercise. Of course, this doesn't mean that they have to be out lifting weights or running marathons, but a daily walk and moving frequently will do wonders for their health, in more ways than one.

At the same time, consider unhealthy food and salt to still be the culprit, and avoid it as much as possible. In the world we live in, eating a low sodium diet isn't at all as hard as it used to be, and there are plenty of options on the market today.

Consistency is key when it comes to the elderly, and the health benefits which arise from this consistency is priceless.

High blood pressure in women:

Although women can easily fit into the unhealthy lifestyle group just as easy as men, there are a few extra factors that can cause high blood pressure in women, and these may require additional care.

- Birth control pills or other hormonal contraceptives can potentially raise a woman's blood pressure.

  Speak with your doctor if you are having trouble with high blood pressure and you are taking any kind of oral contraceptive, as these may easily be related.

- Pregnancy – much the same as when a woman is on birth control, pregnancy will change her hormones, making it much easier for her to suffer from hypertension.

  Developing hypertension from pregnancy is rare when it is compared to all the other ways men and women develop hypertension in their lives, but it still does happen, and it's important to understand what it means when it does.

  When a woman is experiencing hypertension from pregnancy, the treatment will be a little different than when the hypertension is a result of contraceptives.

For the woman who is on contraceptives, there are a variety of options as far as treatment goes. Your doctor may change the method of contraceptive, putting you on something with fewer hormones, or a lower dosage of hormones.

She may also recommend that you make some of the lifestyle changes that I have mentioned already. Cut salt out of your diet as much as possible. Make sure you are a healthy weight. Get daily physical exercise. And, perhaps one of the most important, reduce stress as much as possible.

Treatment for a pregnant mother with hypertension is largely up to the doctor, and it is decided based on a variety of factors. First of all, if the mother is experiencing adverse side effects, he may have her put on an IV.

If the baby is mature enough to be delivered, the decision is made whether to let the child to go full term, or to induce labor and deliver the child early. This decision is based on a variety of factors, and must be discussed between the mother and the doctor.

The only benefit that arises from hormonal/pregnancy induced hypertension is that it will go away whenever the cause is stopped. If a woman were to change her contraceptive plan, or when a mother gives birth to her child, the hypertension generally clears on its own.

However, it is important to note that you must stick with your healthy lifestyle, or you will risk developing it again.

High blood pressure in children:

High blood pressure in children is also rare, but when it does happen, it can be just as serious as high blood pressure in adults. If the child with high blood pressure is under 10 years old, tests are done as this is often indicative of another underlying medical condition.

However, if the child is over 10 years old or is a teenager, lifestyle is often a factor. In this modern world, many children spend more of their time in front of electronics than they do getting exercise, and it does begin to take a toll on their health.

In addition, healthy eating is a constant struggle for the mother of children, as it is a rare thing for them to choose heart healthy foods over junk food.

Yet, just as with adults, many times a child's blood pressure can be brought back down to normal levels through minor lifestyle changes. Healthy eating and daily physical exercise are crucial for a healthy life, regardless of how old an individual is.

These groups can be considered the general groups of society, but they don't cover everyone – what about those who have high blood pressure and are dealing with another medical condition on top of it?

Don't worry, in the next chapter, we are going to examine these special situations.

Chapter 5 – Special Situations

Though much of society can be fit into general groups, there are always going to be special considerations that need to be made for those who are dealing with special circumstances. So what special things must these people to do help with their blood pressure, and what factors causes them to be at greater risk than others?

Studies have shown that approximately 25% of people with Type 1 Diabetes and up to 80% of those with Type 2 Diabetes also have high blood pressure.

Now, when you are a diabetic, you have too much sugar in your blood. This is because your body is unable to process blood sugar properly, which leads to health issues on its own.

A person with Type 1 diabetes produces enough insulin in their blood, but their body is unable to use this insulin. A person with Type 2 diabetes either doesn't produce insulin at all, or doesn't produce enough for the body to use and function properly.

A person with either form of diabetes is already at greater risk for heart attack or stroke.

And sadly, this is not a result of having high blood pressure. When a person has diabetes, they are put at this risk because of the diabetes itself. Then, when they have high blood pressure on top of it, they are put at an even higher risk than they were before.

Doctors who have diabetic patients with hypertension are incredibly careful to keep their blood pressure at a reasonable level. Of course, it is possible to lower your blood pressure too much, though this is rare. Instead, they do everything they can to keep the blood pressure below 130/80, with the bottom number being of extreme importance.

So what can a person in this special situation do? What are the treatment options?

Although diet and lifestyle choices are at the forefront of the treatment, many doctors will also prescribe medication known as ACE inhibitors in an effort to keep blood pressure levels low. Though other blood pressure medication can be used, ACE inhibitors are thought to also work to protect the kidneys, which is crucial for someone with a lot of sugar in their blood and urine.

And what about those people who already have kidney disease, and also develop high blood pressure?

As you may know, there are a variety of different things that can cause kidney disease besides high blood pressure, and a person may end up developing this disease before they are faced with hypertension.

Hypertension that is caused by kidney disease is known as Renal Hypertension, and it must be treated in a special way.

The very first thing a person with renal hypertension must do is examine their lifestyle. Often, alcohol is a factor when it comes to kidney disease, as it is the kidney's job to work with the liver to rid the body of the substance. No matter how much you drink, you need to quit if you have reached this level of problems with your health.

As you have seen already, alcohol is a defining factor in high blood pressure anyway, and if you are adding more on top of the disease you already have, you are only asking for more and more problems. It's time to get completely sober.

More often than not, a person with renal hypertension is given blood pressure medication in an attempt to lower the blood pressure without too much trouble, but with kidney disease, this is not always effect.

In extreme cases, surgery and stenting needs to be performed in the kidneys, helping them to function better – resulting in better filtration of the blood.

As you can imagine, for a person with kidney disease and high blood pressure, diet and exercise are at the forefront of the treatment, along with anything extra that can be done to bring the blood pressure back down. With high blood pressure being a risk factor for kidney disease in the first place, having both at the same time can cause the disease to progress, and may even result in kidney failure.

High blood pressure is a condition that needs to be addressed in anyone who has it, regardless of the age of the individual. However, there are those who need to take extra precaution when it comes to their health.

If you are dealing with multiple health problems, understand that you are not alone, and that you, too, can treat both the hypertension and anything else that is ailing you. It takes some deliberate action on your part, and a lot of cooperation with your doctor, but you will manage to pull through.

First things first. If you are going to get your blood pressure under control before it turns into something worse, or if you are already dealing with that worse thing and are looking to rid yourself of hypertension, too, you are going to need – a plan.

In the next chapter, I am going to show you how to formulate the right plan for you. This will include the things you need to do, the things you need to avoid, and your goals.

Trust me, once you draw up your own plan, sticking with it is going to be easier than you think, and you are going to watch those numbers drop.

Healthy lifestyle, here you come.

Chapter 6 – It's All Part of the Plan

Some people like to plan everything, others like to plan nothing. However, if you are going to get your blood pressure under control and start living this healthy lifestyle, you are going to need to have something to aim for. This doesn't have to be a long dissertation of all your hopes and dreams, but it should contain what you wish to accomplish in your journey.

Grab a pen and paper, right now, then sit down and analyze what you have been doing that has given you high blood pressure.

This is sort of a moment of self-reflection, in which you get to determine what choices you have made that have brought you to where you are today. This may be fun, or it may be painful, but it is necessary in order for you to make a change.

Be honest with yourself here. Of course, nobody likes to write down that they now have health problems because they ate a poor diet, or because they were inactive, but it is these realizations that will help you change, and not make the same mistakes again in the future.

You don't have to be incredibly detailed in what you write, but you do have to be incredibly honest. What was it that you did that brought you here today?

After you have identified what you have been doing, write down the things you need to change.

Again, you don't have to be overly detailed, but you do need to get the point across to yourself that you need to make a change. Perhaps this needs to be something drastic – write down that you are now going to quit smoking.

Perhaps it needs to be a little more subtle – write down that you are going to cut back on the amount of salt you have been eating.

I can't tell you exactly what you need to say, because it is personal. Instead, focus on what you want to change, what you need to change, and how it's going to help your blood pressure come back down to a normal level – and give you your healthy life back.

Now, it's going to get a little bit harder. You have identified the things you need to change, now you are going to write down *how you are going to change them.*

At this point, you do need to be detailed. If you are going to give up a bad habit, write down how you are going to do that. Perhaps you are going to get a support group to help you change. Perhaps you are going to wean yourself off of it, or perhaps you are going to walk away from it and never look back.

It doesn't matter how you go about making this change, as long as you really do. If you are going to change an inactive lifestyle, write down how you plan to do that – write down that you are interested in doing, and what you would like to accomplish. Again, this can be a painful thing to do, but it doesn't have to be. You can be happy about the change, and hopeful for the futures. As I said, this could be one of the best things that has happened to you, if it puts you on track for a healthy life.

After you write down how you are going to change, write down what your goals are for making these changes.

At this point, you can go back to being as vague or as detailed as you want. You can write down something like what you hope to weight at the end of six months, or you can write down that you wish to be happy spending time with the people you love.

You can write down something as basic as you want your blood pressure to be brought back down to a normal level. Whatever your goals are in making this change, write it down in as much or as little detail as you want.

You now have the issue, the solution, and what you are going to get from that solution. For the final thing, you are going to write down why you are making this decision.

One of the biggest points of having a plan is to keep yourself motivated in the long run. With this final point, write down why you are going to make the change. It can be a reason that has everything to do with you, or it can be a reason that has nothing to do with you.

You can say something like, *I'm doing this for my kids.*

Or, *I'm doing this for my grandkids.*

Or, *I'm doing this for myself, because I am worth it.*

As long as you write down something that is going to inspire you to stick with your plan every time you see it, write it down. There is no wrong answer, all you need to write is an honest answer.

Next, take your plan and either post it somewhere you can see it often, or fold it up and keep it where you can look back over it whenever you want.

That's your plan, now let's put it into motion.

Chapter 7 – Welcome to the DASH Diet

As you well know, the first thing your doctor looked at when he diagnosed you with hypertension is the lifestyle you are living. Though this does include exercise, stress, and dealing with bad habits such as smoking and drinking alcohol, perhaps the greatest thing your doctor was interested in was what you are eating.

The typical American diet is filled with fats, sugars, refined carbs, and most of all – salt. It seems there can't be a family dinner without the salt being passed around the table and showered over every plate in the area. It's true, salt does enhance the flavors of food, but in the long run, it's not doing anyone any favors.

With over 3 million new cases of hypertension being diagnosed every year, doctors had dieticians alike have worked together to create an eating plan that will help lower high blood pressure, while still allowing you to eat many of the same foods you have always loved.

This diet has come to be known as the DASH diet.

When the Dash diet was first introduced to the public, it was quickly proven to lower blood pressure every bit as well as many of the medications on the market, even allowing the participants to eat as much as 3300mg of salt per day.

Intrigued, many scientists began running studies on the DASH diet, and have concluded that it is capable of reducing the risk of heart disease, stroke, kidney disease, and even some cancers. Of course, it wasn't long before men and women alike got on board with the diet for weight loss – which it also proved incredibly effective for.

The DASH diet works as a cycle. If you are using it to lower your blood pressure, you are going to also lose weight. If you are using it to lose weight, you are also going to lower your blood pressure. It's a complete win all around.

So what is the DASH diet exactly?

Originally, the DASH diet focused primarily on white pastas, but that was largely due to the time in which it was introduced. Over the years, the DASH diet has been refined to a much healthier standard, and now is an excellent aid to start a healthy lifestyle.

Unlike the low carb diets, the DASH diet allows for carbs, but only the healthy kind. No white, processed, refined anything. Instead you are going to eat Whole grain, whole wheat, vegetables, fruits and plenty of protein. Of course, there is room for the fats, too, but not nearly so many fats as the standard American diet.

The DASH diet is also careful to cut back on both salt and sugar – especially the refined sugars. Anything that is white, bleached, and refined is not allowed on this diet, as those are empty calories that spike your blood sugar and are converted into fats.

One of the main benefits of the DASH diet is that is has been developed to be flexible. It doesn't matter what your preference is (vegan, vegetarian, carnivore) you are going to find a variation that works for you.

It's also important to note that this is not a restricting diet by any means. If you follow the meal plan, you will see that you are allowed more than enough food throughout the day, so there is never a need to feel deprived or hungry.

But what does a typical day on the DASH diet look like?

Though you can adjust for your own personal needs, this is what the standard DASH day looks like. Remember to get your groups from a variety of sources, so you are getting all the nutrition you need, as well as keeping things interesting.

Whole grain servings: 6-12

Fruit servings: 4-6

Vegetable servings: 4-6

Low fat or non-fat dairy or dairy substitute servings: 2-4

Lean meat, fish, lean protein sources servings: 1.5-2.5

Nuts, seeds, and legume servings: 3-6 per week

Fats and sweets servings: 2-4 (make sure they are extremely limited)

Though right now you might be used to eating bacon and eggs whenever you feel like it, you need to realize that there is a healthier way of eating that is better for your body in a number of ways.

The more you embrace this healthy way of eating, the better you are going to feel, and the sooner you are going to see those numbers drop – both for your blood pressure and on the scale.

You know what whole grains and fruits and vegetables are, and you know how to select lean proteins that you enjoy eating. Use the DASH diet as you eating plan, and enjoy everything as you once did, just in a healthier way. Remember to ditch the salt and the refined sugars, and focus on eating real, whole foods.

As I said, it doesn't matter what your motive is to get on this diet, whether you are doing it for the sake of weight loss, or if you are doing it simply for the sake of your blood pressure. Once you get on this diet – and after you have stayed with it for a week or two, you are going to see the benefits start rolling in.

DASH all the way to a healthy new life.

Chapter 8– The Lazy Person's Guide to Blood Pressure Exercises

I know, I know – exercising is the last thing you want to have to do on top of everything else you are already dealing with. But, with high blood pressure, it is crucial for you to get in shape and bring those numbers back down.

One thing few people think about as they are deciding on a workout regimen is that their normal lives are supposed to be carrying on in spite of all of this. Your boss may be sympathetic to your situation, but he's still going to expect you to be at work and get your job done.

Your children may not understand why you are feeling way that you do, or they may understand that something isn't right and wish they knew what it was, but that isn't going to change the fact that you need to be up and taking care of them and your other daily duties whenever the need arises.

So, when choosing the right exercise regimen for yourself you need to find something that you enjoy, as well as something that is going to fit into your busy schedule.

Start off with mind exercises and guided meditation.

Countless research studies have proven that meditation cures a variety of ailments, including anxiety, depression, and stress. If you are dealing with high stress, and you just can't seem to catch a break, try meditating every morning.

With dozens if not hundreds of resources online, you can choose the meditation style that is right for you, as well as where you watch it. YouTube has many different guided mediations ranging from only 10 minutes to several hours long. Depending on how much time you have and what your personal needs are, you can select the meditation, press play, and forget everything else in the world while your stress is swept away.

The more often you practice, the less stress you will have. This, as you know, is going to have a direct impact on your blood pressure level.

Do something that relaxes you at least a couple time per week.

In this modern world, we all tend to overextend ourselves and live hectic lives. Although we do this with the intention of getting as much done as possible, it does tend to take a toll on our health as time passes.

In order to lower your blood pressure, you are going to have to relieve some of this stress. Make a deliberate effort to do something you find relaxing at least a couple times per week, every week. It doesn't have to be anything big or elaborate, and it could be something as simple as looking through your favorite magazine or reading a good book.

As long as you are doing something that reduces the stress in your life and leaves you feeling good when you are done, do it.

As you have seen already, stress is one of the biggest causes of high blood pressure, so reducing stress as much as possible is going to have a direct – and significant – effect on bringing your blood pressure back down to a normal and healthy level.

Add cardio in at least 3 times per week.

When it comes to doing cardio, things can easily get too crazy too soon. Just because you are working out, it doesn't mean that you have to do something that you don't enjoy. Cardio is anything that gets your heart rate up – and this can be done in a way you enjoy.

Getting your heartrate up is the most important thing you can do for your body at this point. If you have a specific goal weight (or weight range) in mind, even better. But, for now, as long as you are getting your heart rate up for at least 20 – 30 minutes per day several times per week, you are going to be helping your blood pressure.

The key to finding a cardio routine that you can stick with is finding something that you enjoy doing.

This can be anything as simple as a walk in the park or around the neighborhood, or something as adventurous as joining a kickboxing or dance class. Just find what makes you happy, find something that you can look forward to doing, and get out there and do it.

Build a support group, and perhaps find a friend that is willing to do the work with you, and you'll have something else that will help you reduce your stress in life, too.

Remember to take a day to rest.

As ironic as it sounds to have a day of rest in a chapter of exercises, it's important that you do take the time to regroup and let your body heal. This is especially important if you haven't been exercising and are now adding it into your day.

Our bodies, while they are meant to serve the purpose we wish for them to serve, are designed to function habitually. This is why you always begin to crave certain things at certain times in the day, even if you are just craving it because of the time of day it is.

As you break out of the inactive lifestyle, your body is going to need time to adjust, and don't be surprised if you don't see your blood pressure numbers drop as you would like at first. When you first begin exercising, you are going to send your body into a mild state of shock which will, in turn, cause it to put on the brakes.

But, with steady practice, and with a determination to advance, your body will begin to change to meet the new requirements you are putting onto it. This is going to include however much fitness you want to achieve, however much weight you want to lose, and however far you want your goals to be.

Set the standard high for yourself at first, then break this standard down into smaller goals and work to achieve them. This is going to help you keep your eyes on the long term prize, but give you the opportunity to celebrate the small victories along the way.

All the while, you will see your blood pressure begin to drop, then gradually – perhaps once a week or so, you can check it to see where it has ended up. Though it is going to take some time – nothing with your health happens overnight – you are going to see it drop further and further, until you have brought it back down to where it should be.

Remember that exercise, along with any other change you make to your body, should be done under the supervision of a doctor. If you are dealing with any of the special circumstances that we have looked at in previous chapters, check with your doctor before beginning any exercise regimen.

Though doctors strongly encourage exercising, if you are pregnant, a diabetic, elderly, or have any special case, it is incredibly important that you get the clear on what you can do before you begin.

The last thing you need to do is cause yourself more problems than what you are dealing with already.

Now take a look at the goals you have written down, and reach for the stars!

Only the sky is the limit.

Chapter 9 – Blood Pressure Management: Your Stress Free Life

Once you fully understand the risks of having hypertension, and you decide to make a change, you have a long journey ahead of you. But, as you work through changing your diet, adopting a new exercise regimen, and quitting harmful habits, you slowly transition into a new part of the journey: management.

As I said before, when many people hear the word "management" when it comes to their health, they begin to think they have something truly wrong with them, and it can have a negative impact on their lives.

The truth about hypertension is that you either have it, or you don't. The numbers will tell you the truth about whether or not you currently have it, and you won't always have it.

With that being said, however, once you have high blood pressure, you will always be at risk for developing it again. Lifestyle will have a direct impact on the likelihood of you developing this again in your lifetime, which is why management is key.

Many people who have been diagnosed with hypertension will make the changes they need to make for a while, but eventually, the old habits begin to creep back in, and the numbers begin to slowly climb back up.

Don't misunderstand, I know that there is no "one size fits all" plan when it comes to the management of anything. There are going to be people who respond well to the treatment, and there are going to be those who don't and need to find something a little different.

There are going to be those who do respond well, but who don't enjoy the treatment and would benefit from changing it slightly to make it more bearable for them.

As you go through your hypertension journey, it's important that you find what works for you. This is why I have outlined different kinds of exercises, and different kinds of foods. Find the one that makes you happy, and the one that brings your blood pressure down to where it should be, and you will be far more likely to stay on the treatment – and be happy with it.

Your health and your happiness are priceless. Work with the methods I have outlined to find what works for you. I guarantee you will find something that you can both stick with in the long run, and enjoy.

As you know by now, there are certain factors that will automatically predispose you to having hypertension, but the lifestyle choices you make are going to far outweigh any of the predispositions you have.

Just because something is in your family line, it doesn't mean that you are doomed to get it yourself, it merely means that you are at a higher risk of developing it in your lifetime.

The most important thing you must understand when it comes to high blood pressure is that the risks that are associated with the condition (all the things we looked at in chapter 2) are only risk factors when your blood pressure is currently high.

If you make every effort to keep your blood pressure low, you can remind yourself that you are also keeping your risk factor for heart attack, stroke, and kidney disease at a lower level as well.

Follow the DASH diet, and remember to exercise regularly. Avoid doing the harmful things that increase your risk factor, and you will find that maintaining a healthy blood pressure range isn't nearly as intimidating as you once thought.

Just remember, as you live your healthy life, you are going to have to monitor where your blood pressure numbers are. This is the only way you will know for sure whether you need to adjust what you are doing.

As you focus on maintaining a healthy level of blood pressure, keep in mind that there are some things that can affect your reading, giving you a false result.

When you go in to have your blood pressure measured, take the necessary steps to get an accurate reading from the doctor or from the machine.

- Do not smoke for at least 2 hours before having your blood pressure measured

- Do not drink coffee or any other caffeinated beverage for at least 2 hours before having your blood pressure measured

- Do not engage in any vigorous activity before having your blood pressure measured

- Relieve yourself in a restroom before going in to have your blood pressure measured

To know without a doubt that you are living the healthy life you need to be, and that it's working, you will need to know for sure you are getting accurate readings. Of course, the only way to do that is to take the time to prepare for your measurements before you have them done.

At first, watching the numbers fluctuate or stay the same can be intimidating. You try everything to bring them down to a normal level, and despite all your hard work they stay the same. But then, the next week when you go in to have your blood pressure measured, it's dropped a few numbers on both ends.

Though there is no way to tell for sure what your blood pressure is going to be when you walk in to have it measured, if you are consistent and careful to live the healthy lifestyle I have outlined, you are going to see those numbers drop.

As you have seen throughout the pages of this book, hypertension is no laughing matter. If it is left untreated, it can result in many devastating conditions and illnesses, which could change your life forever.

Living a life with as little stress as possible is crucial for ridding yourself of hypertension and bringing your blood pressure down to a normal level.

Don't forget to get outside and do the things you enjoy. Spend time with the people you love, doing the things you love to do. Yes, diet and exercise are going to play a crucial role in your healing, but don't forget what I said about stress.

You deserve to live a happy and healthy life, so let whatever is stressing you out go, and live life like you ought to.

Good luck!

Conclusion

There you have it, everything you need to know about high blood pressure, and how you can bring yours back under control. I hope this book was able to show you exactly what you need to do to lower your blood pressure and live a healthy lifestyle you can actually enjoy.

Health is an all important thing, and all too many people take theirs for granted. They eat what they want, do what they want, and refuse to take care of themselves, without realizing the dangers they are putting themselves in.

As you have seen, once some of the side effects occur, they can be permanently damaging or even fatal. It's important that you get your blood pressure under control, and that you do it as soon as possible.

I hope this book was also able to inspire you to take the steps you need to take to bring your blood pressure down to where it needs to be. It can be intimidating at first, but with time, perseverance, and patience, you will see those numbers drop, and you'll start to feel better in no time.

Shake off that feeling of despondency and get excited for these changes. You are doing not only yourself a favor, but your family, friends, and loved ones. Every step you take to live a happier and healthier life, the better off you are in the long run.

I hope this book was able to show you all the alternatives you can make to enjoy life as much as you did before, and that you get out there and show you friends and family what it means to be happy and healthy, all wrapped into one.

Be the inspiration they need to also live a healthy life, and break the cycle of high blood pressure for good.

It only takes one person to make a real difference, and by changing your own lifestyle, you can make a real impact on society. Now get out there and live your healthy life with a passion.

You've still got a lot of fight left – use it to show the world what you're made of.

Good luck!

Made in United States
North Haven, CT
20 July 2023

39302303R00032